Mandalas Coloring Book for Children
Kids Fun Drawing Magical Beautiful

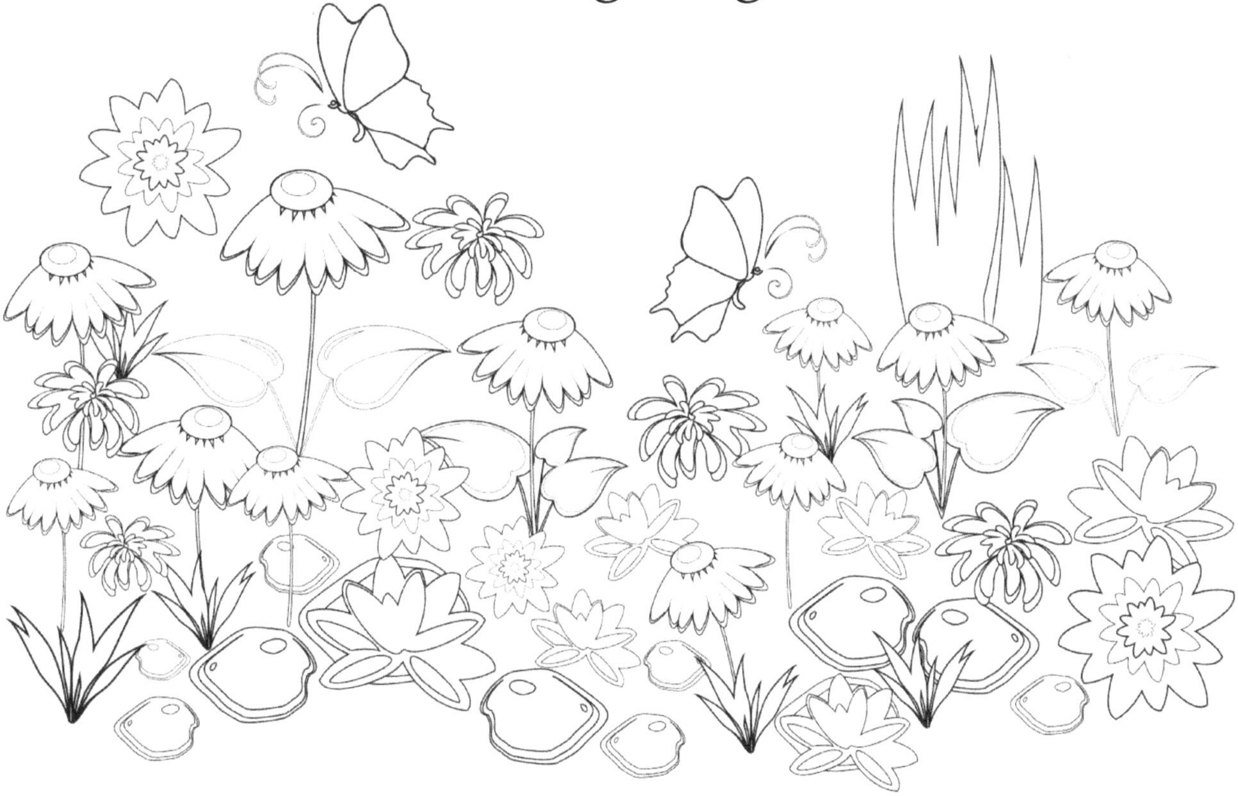

Annie Jr.

Mandalas Coloring Book for Children Kids Fun Drawing Magical Beautiful

ISBN-13: 978-1533280718

ISBN-10: 1533280711

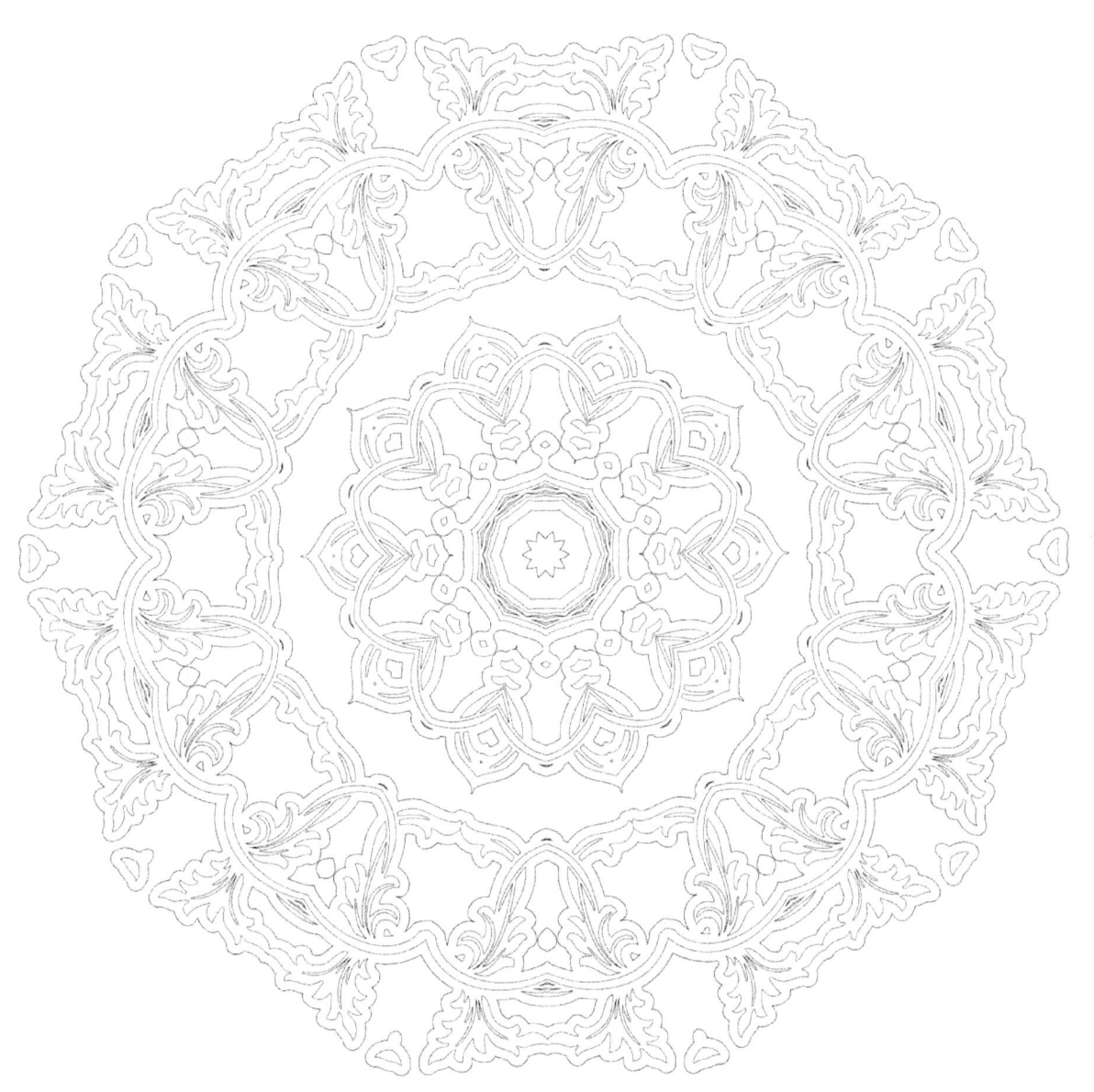

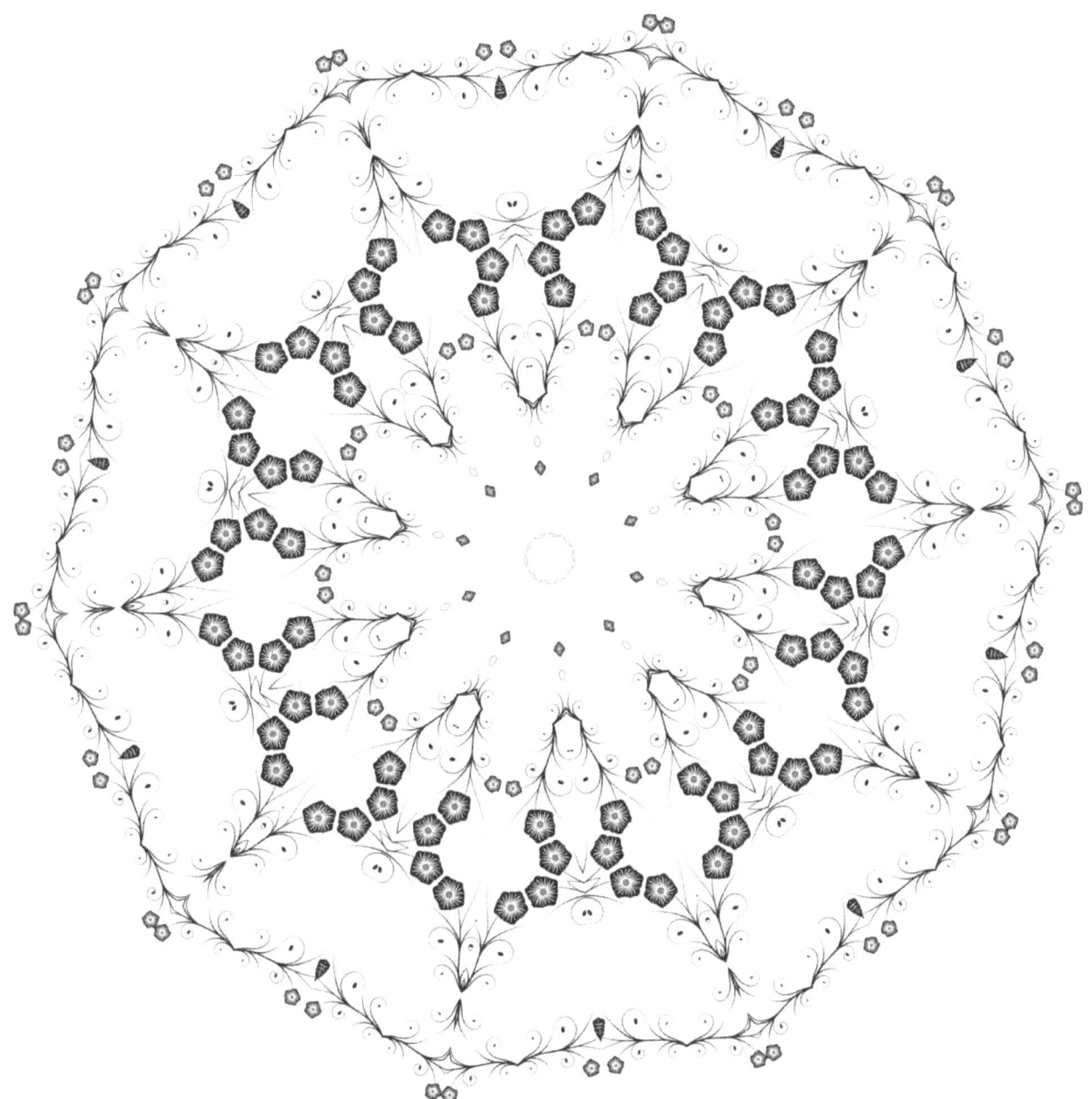

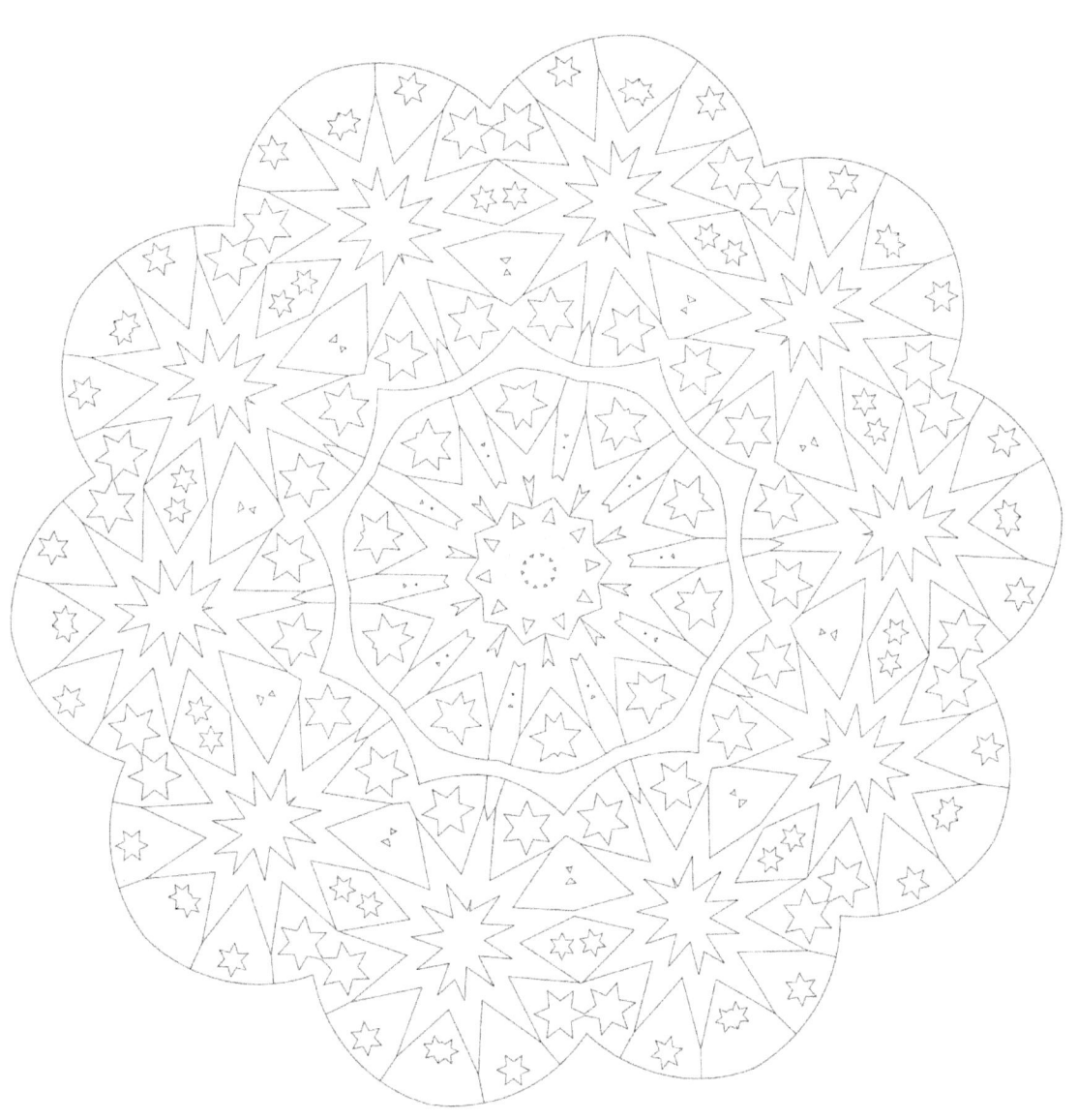

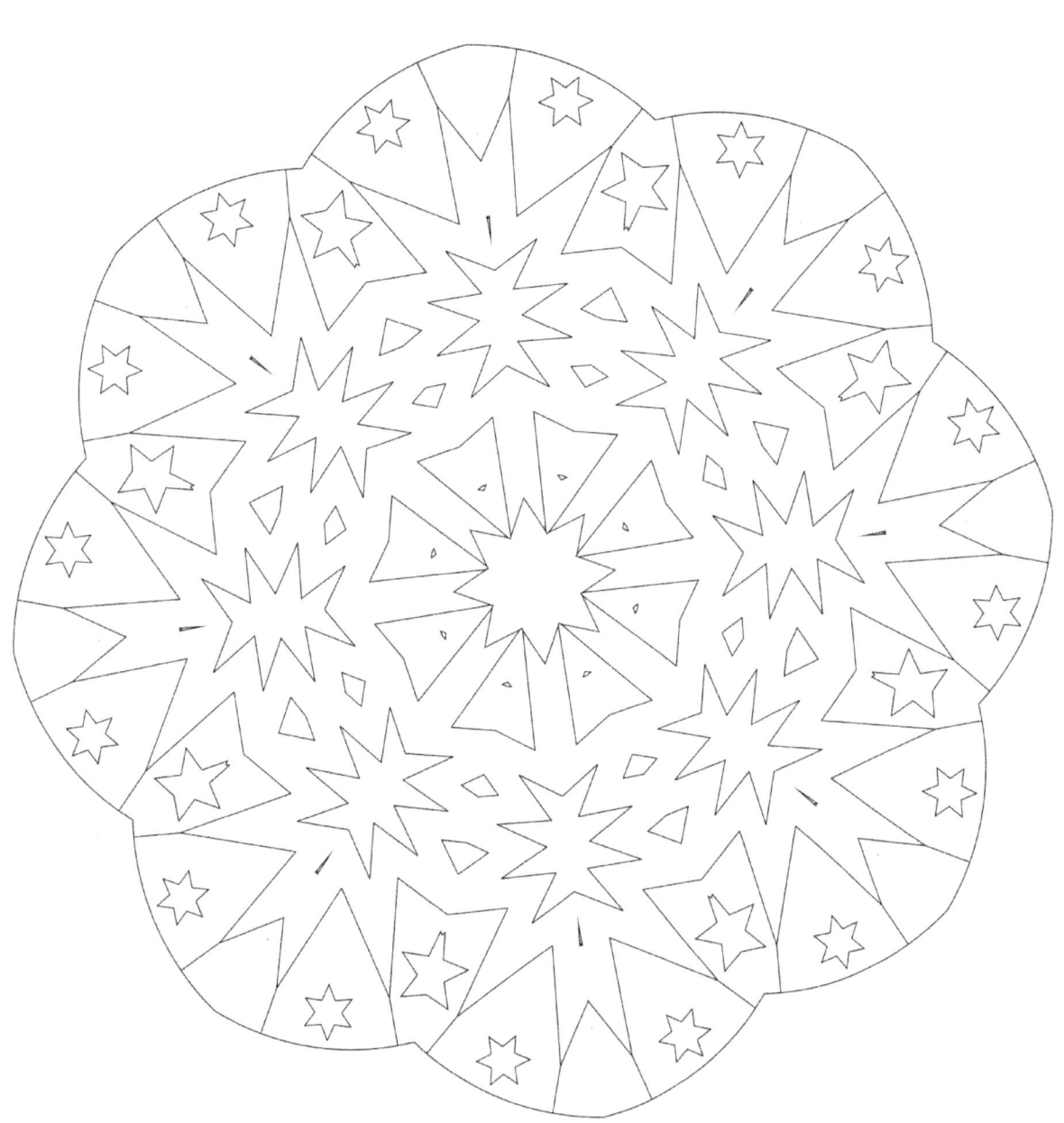

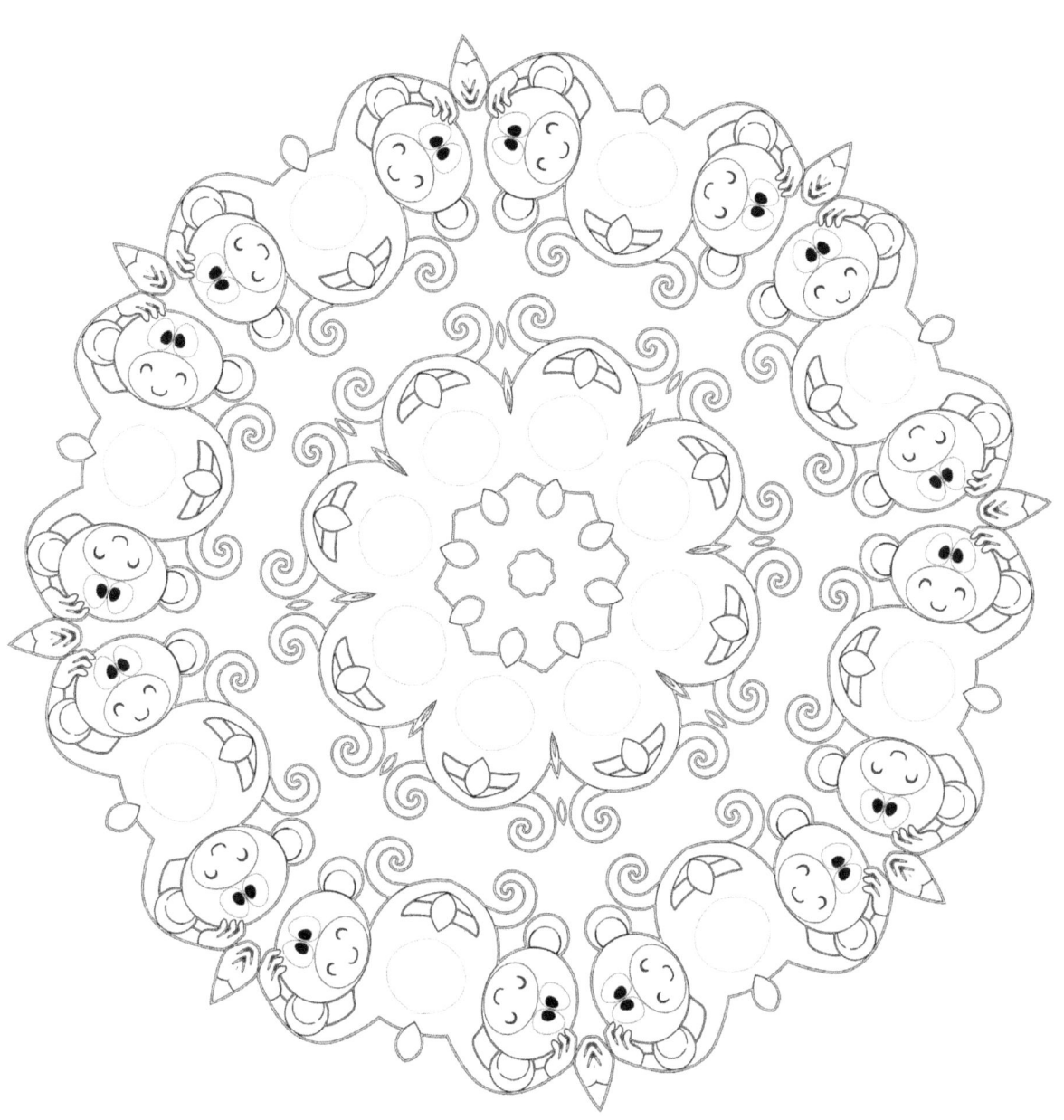

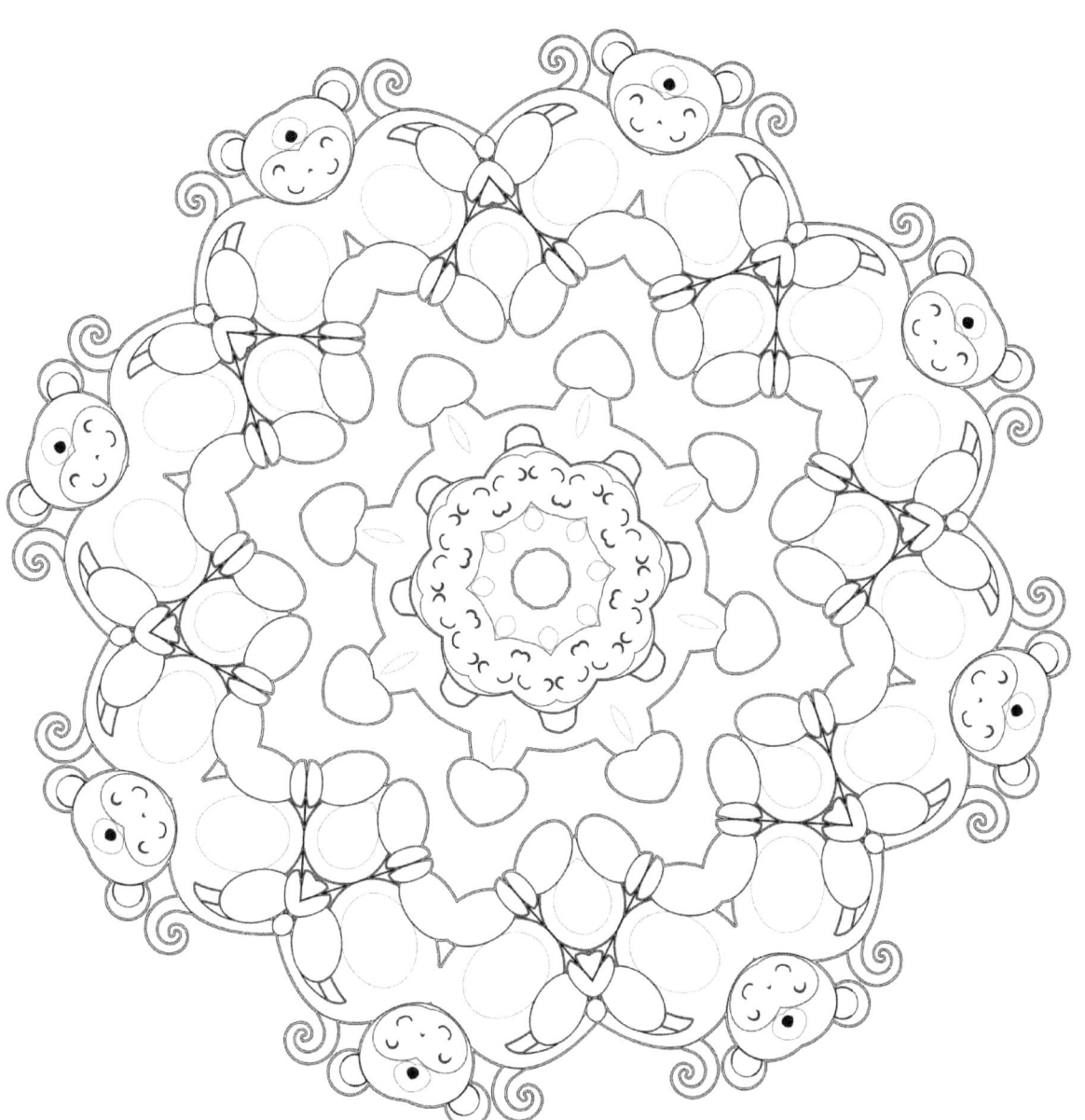

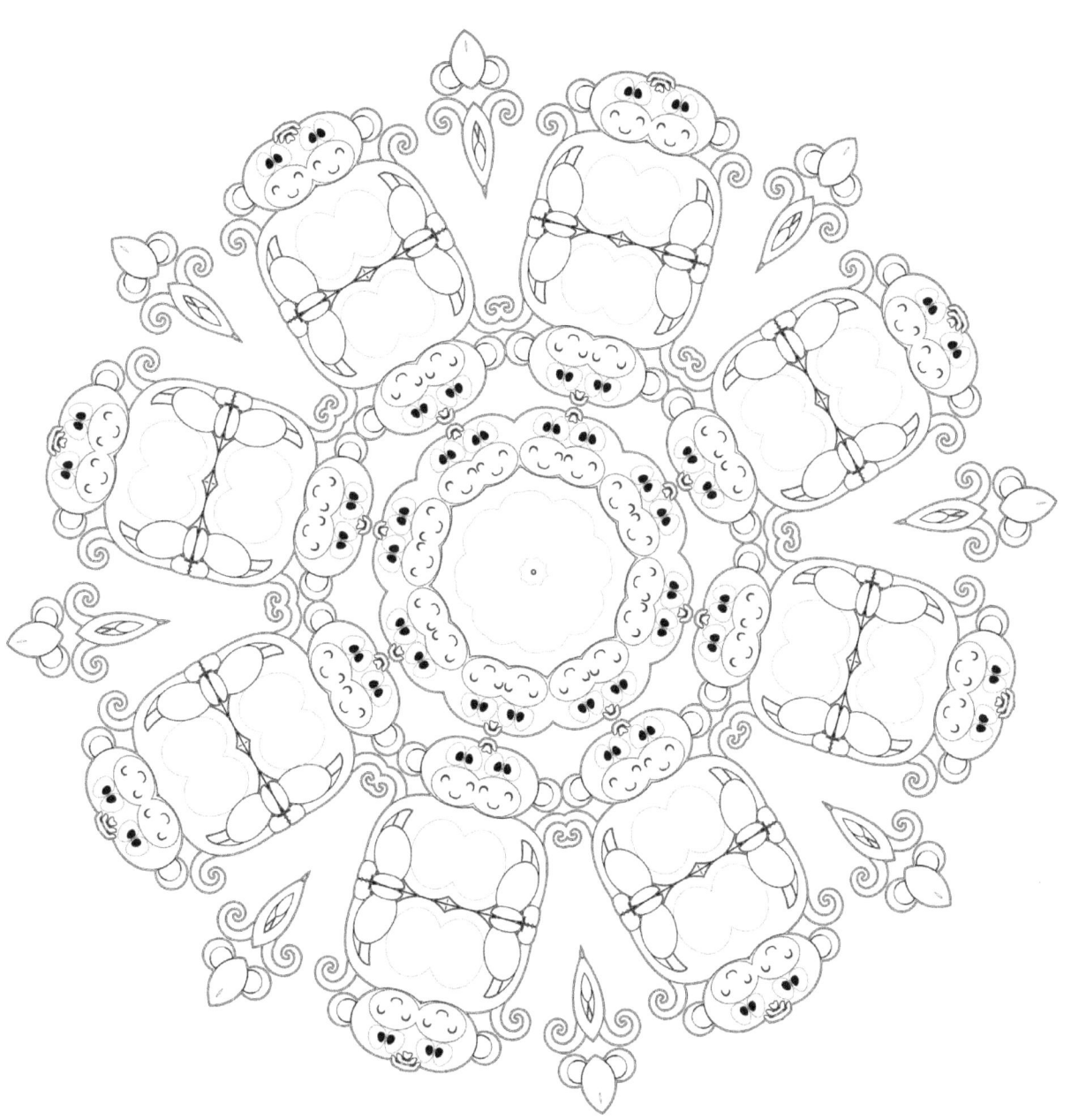

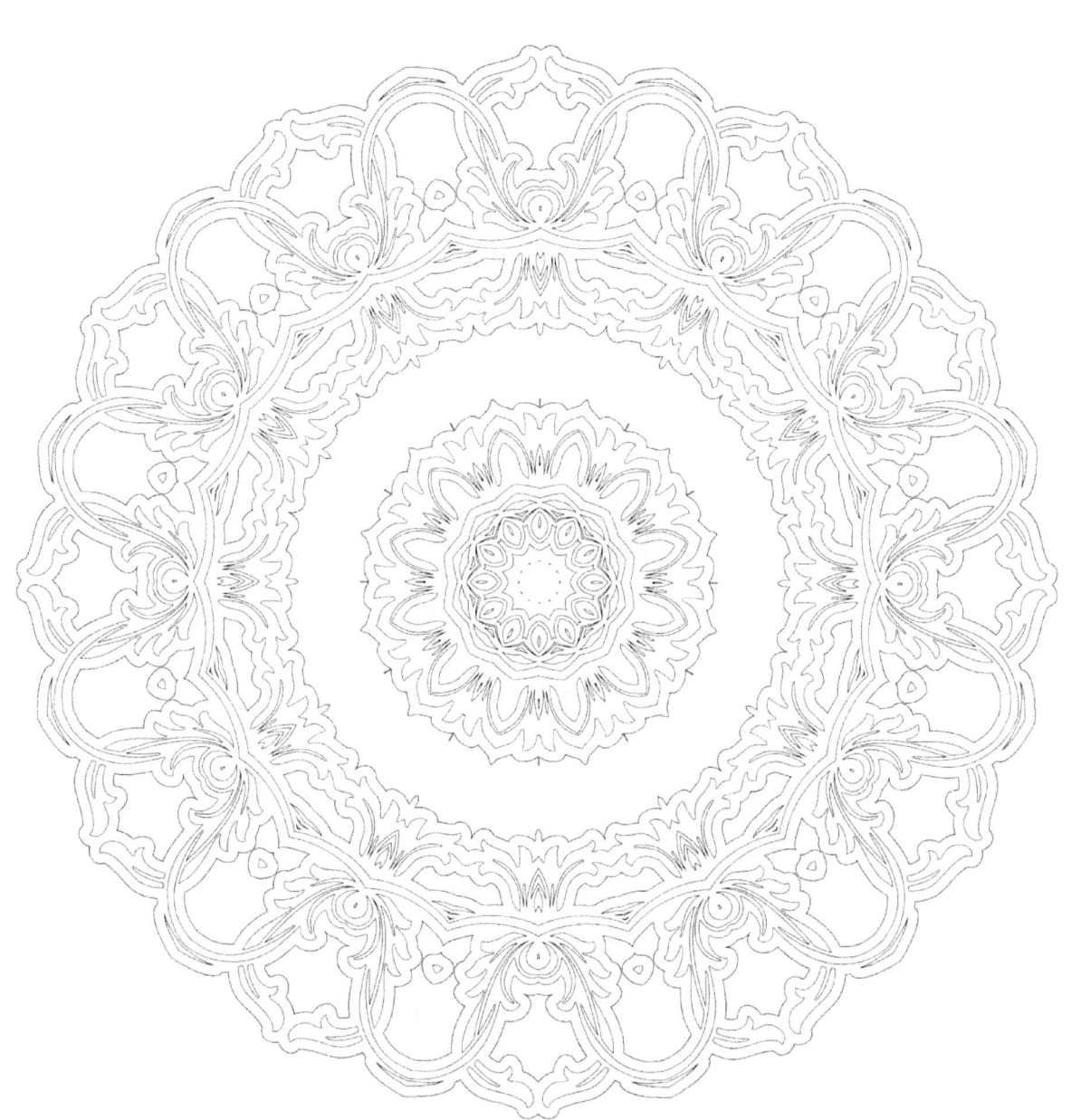

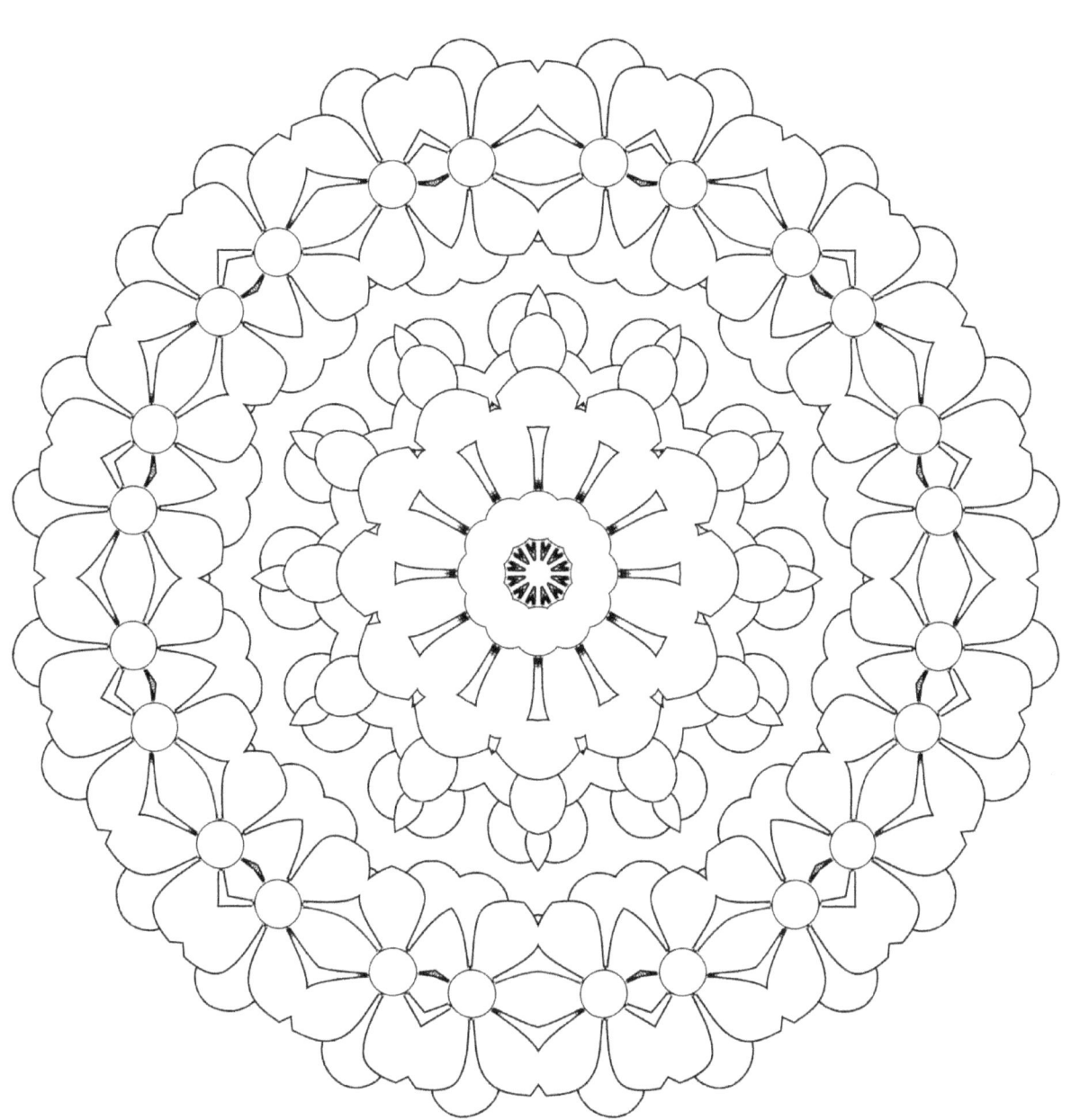

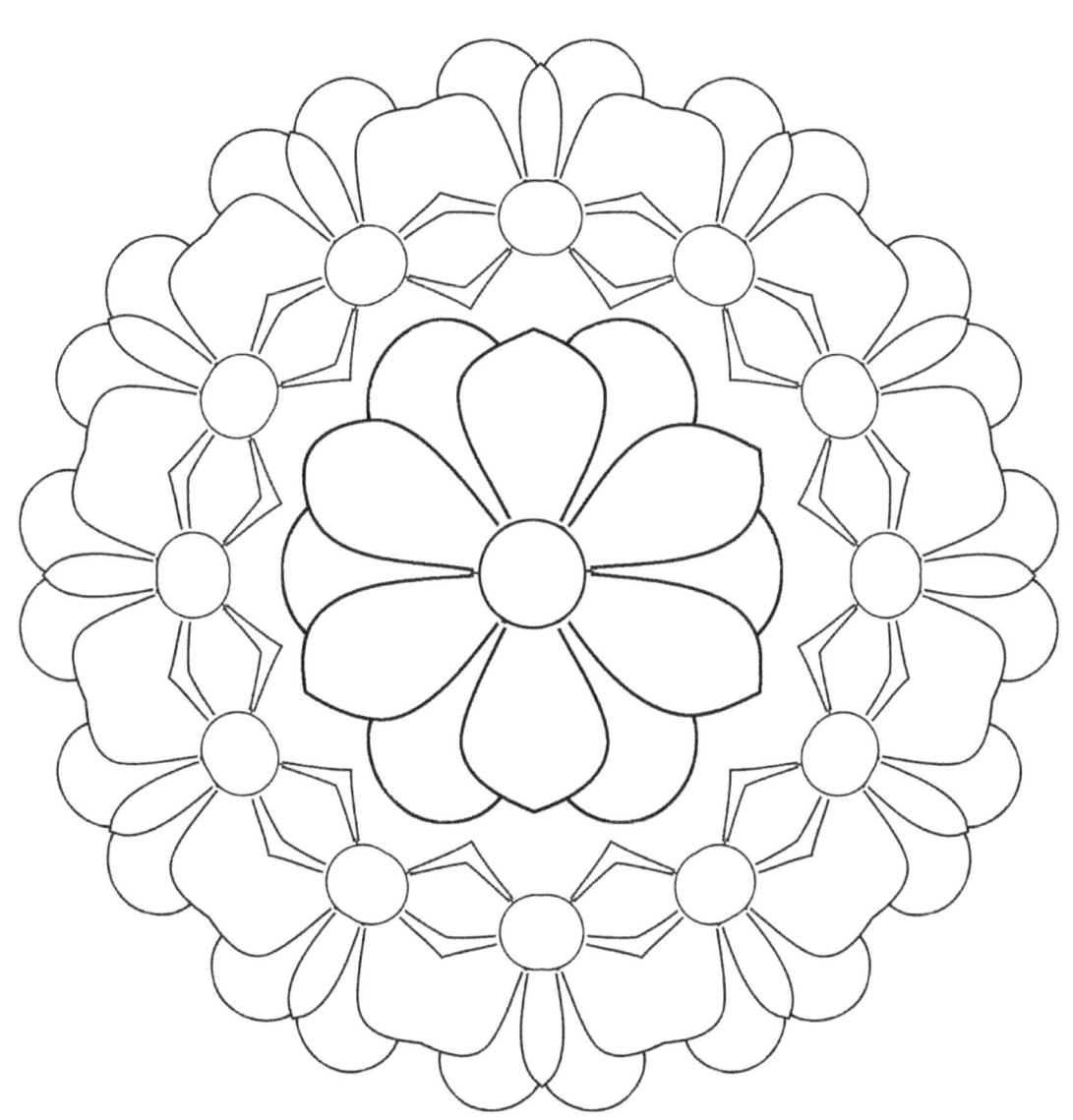

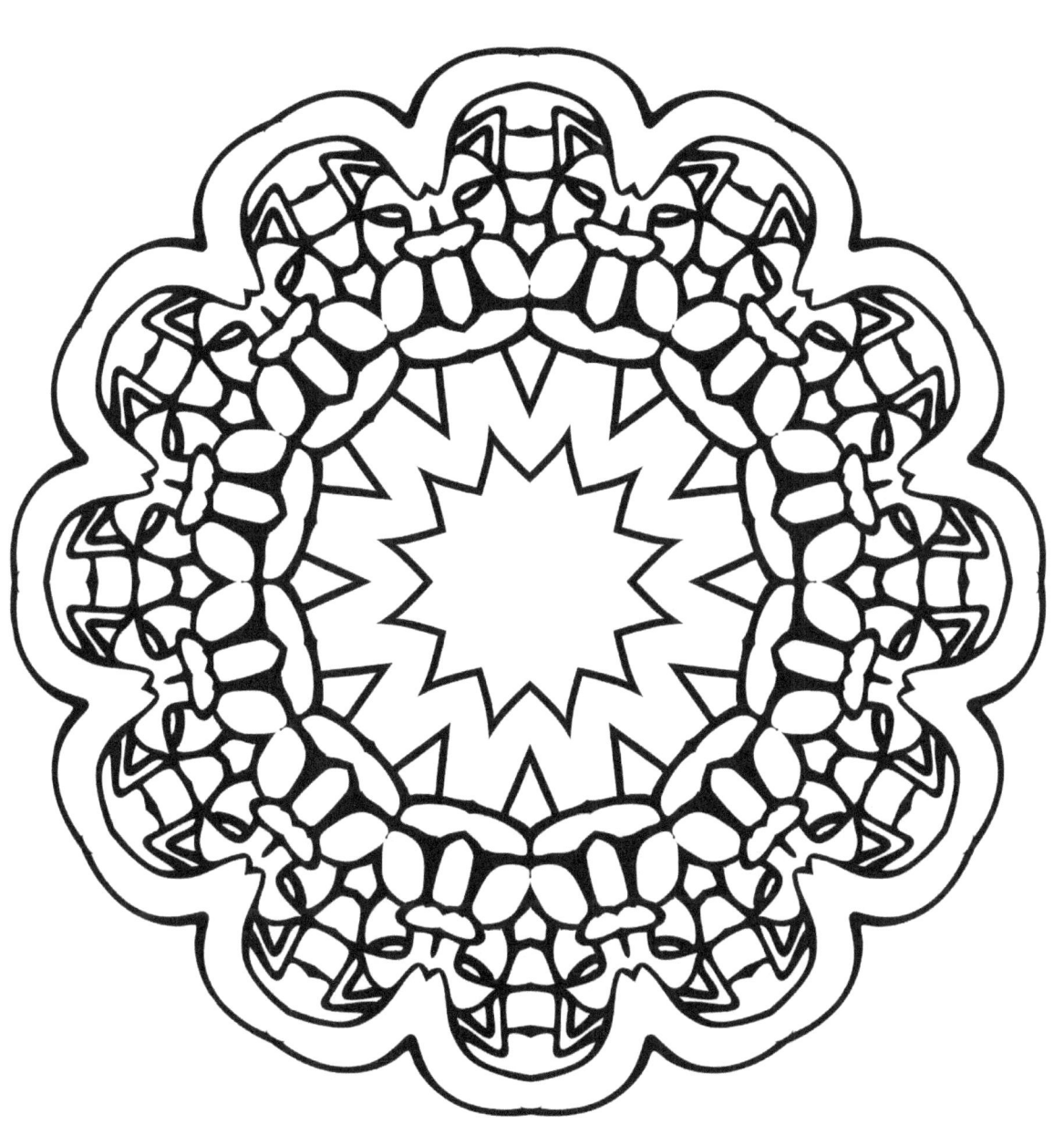

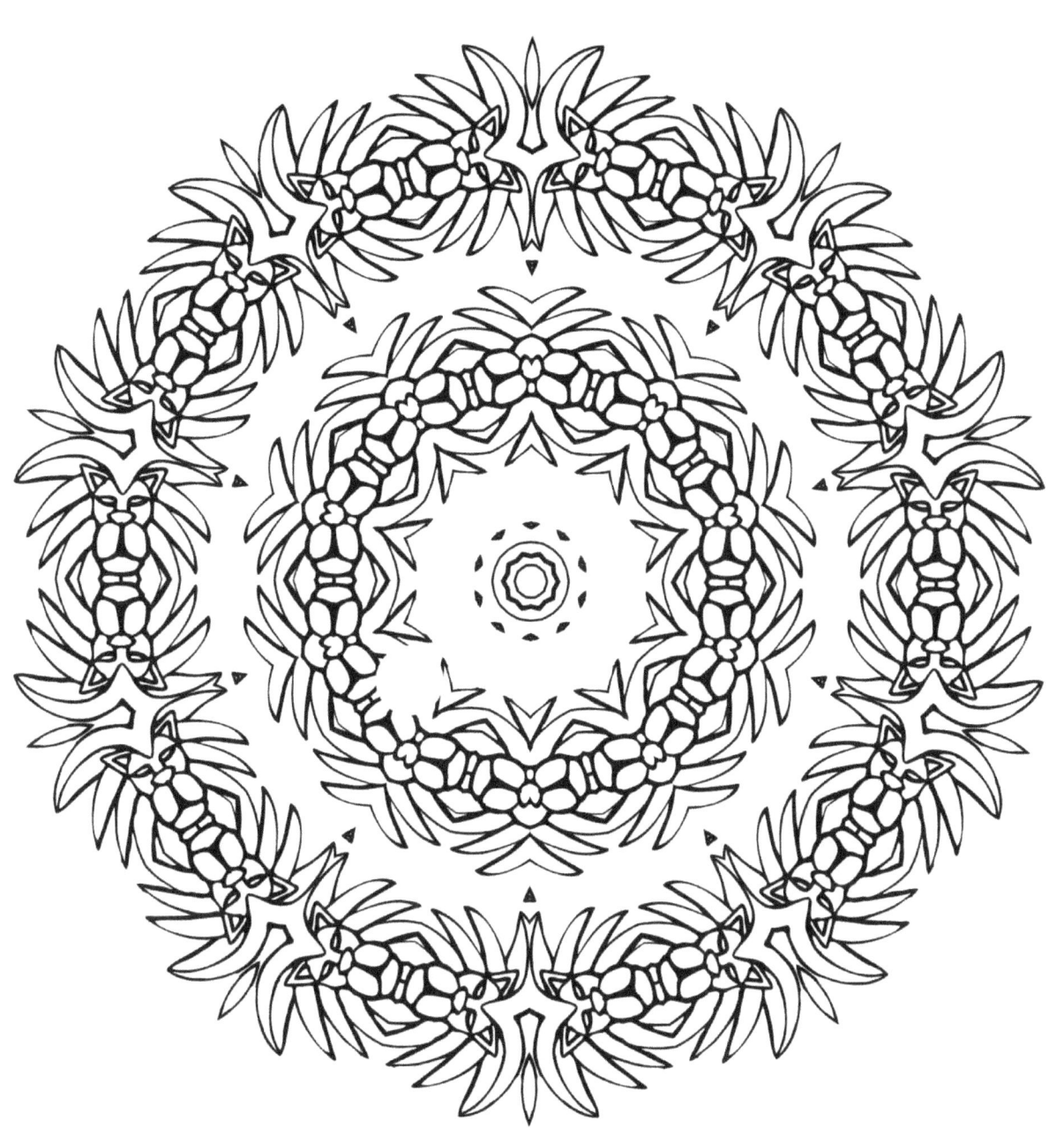

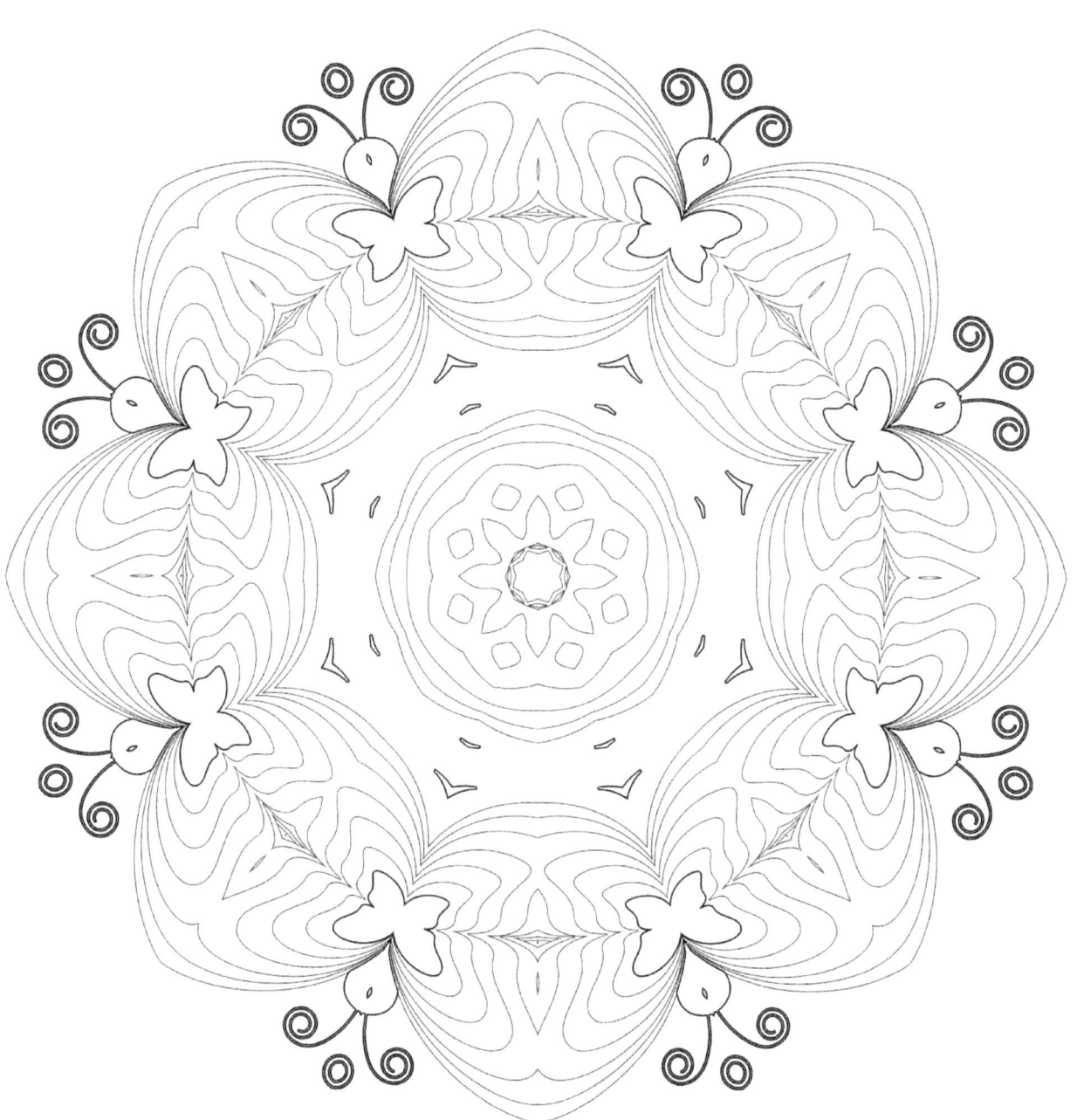

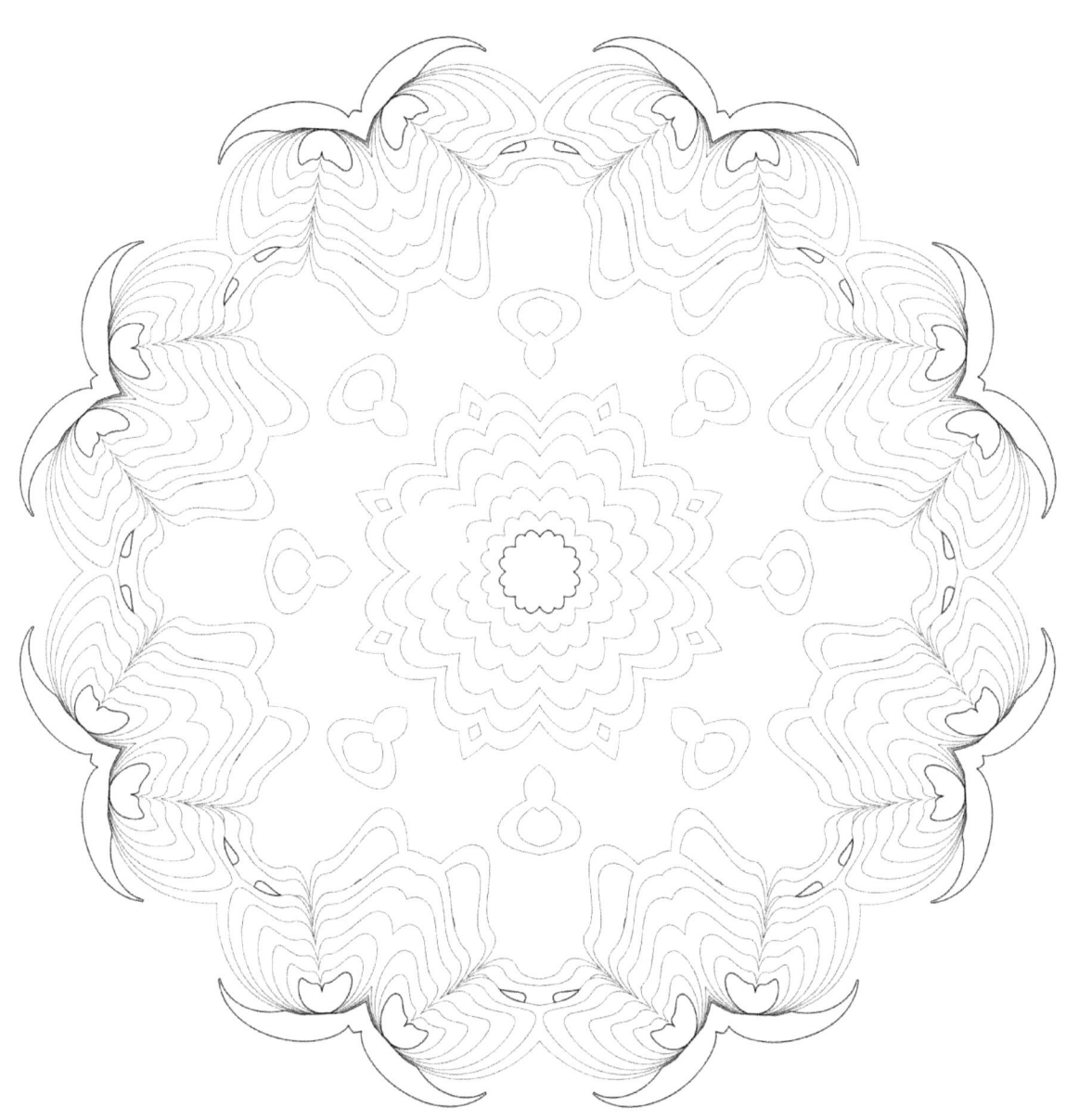

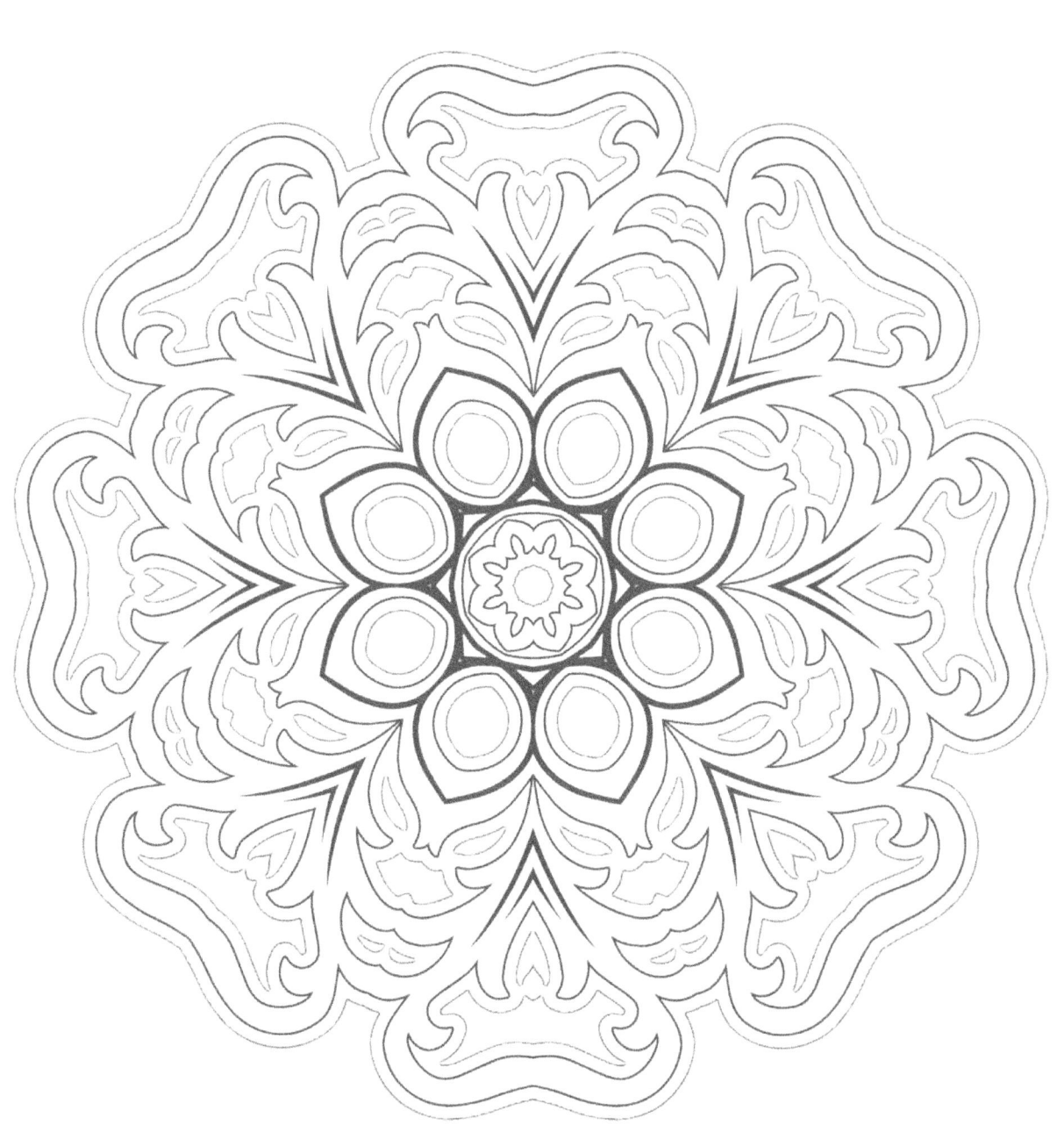

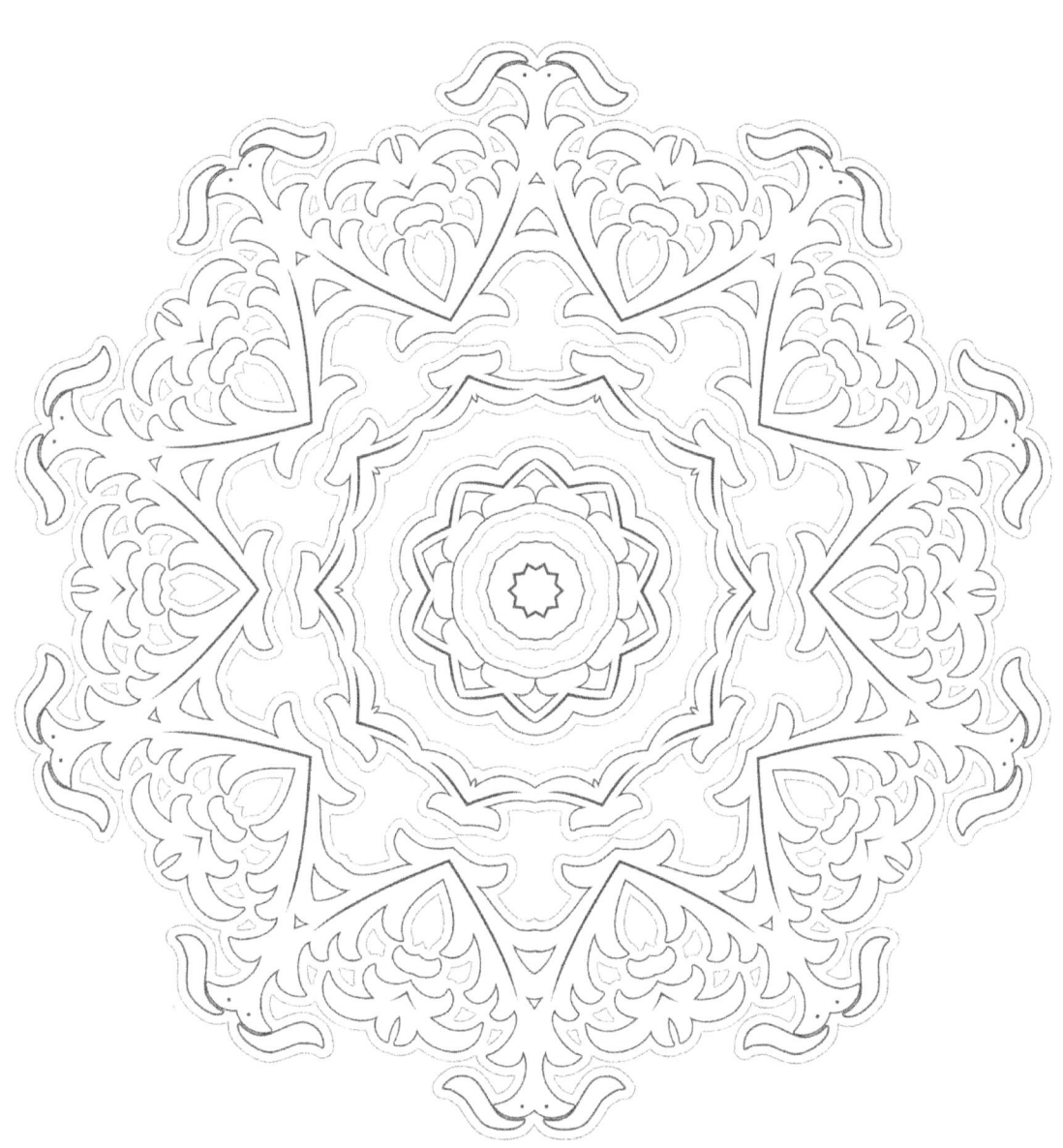

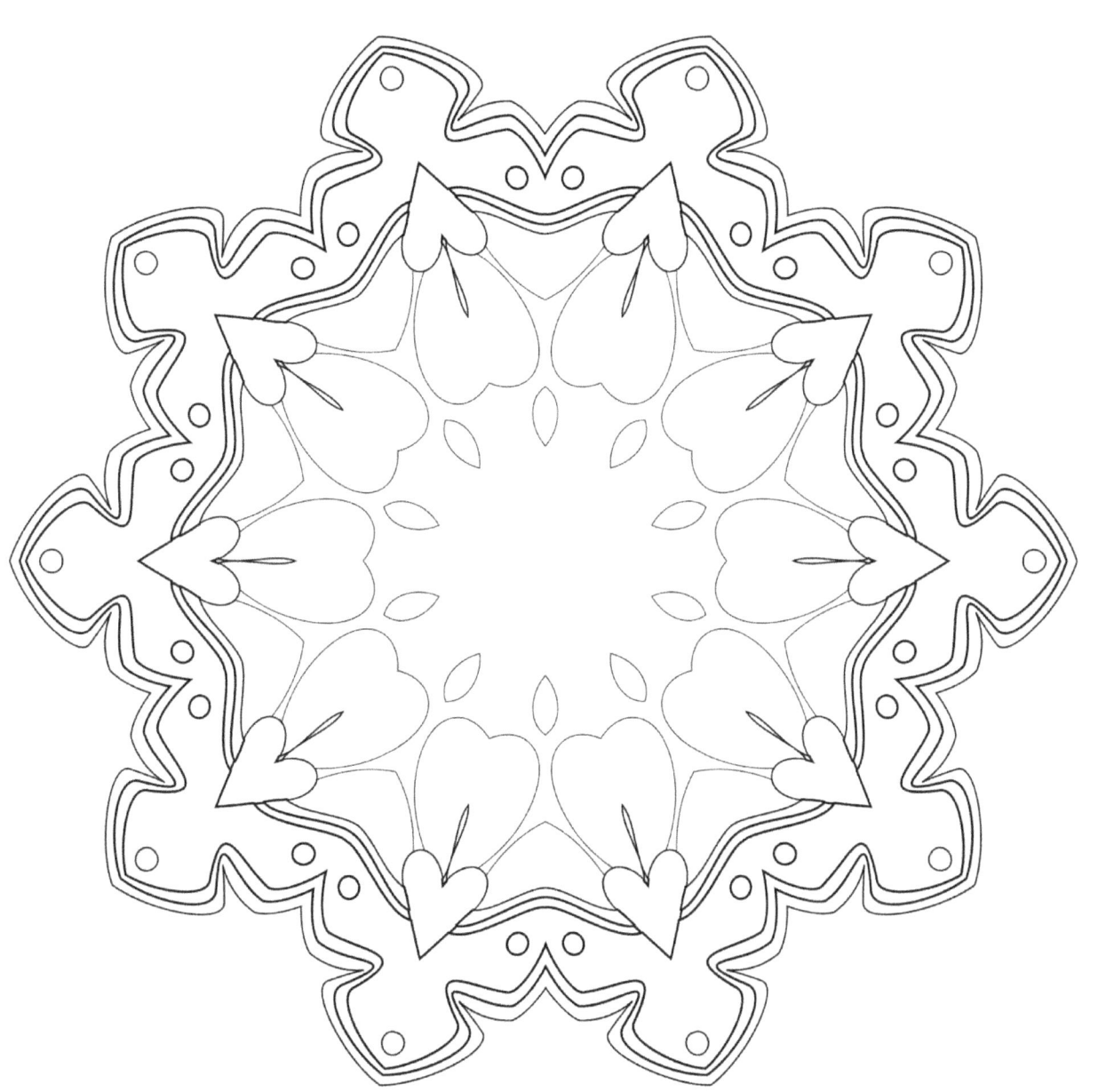

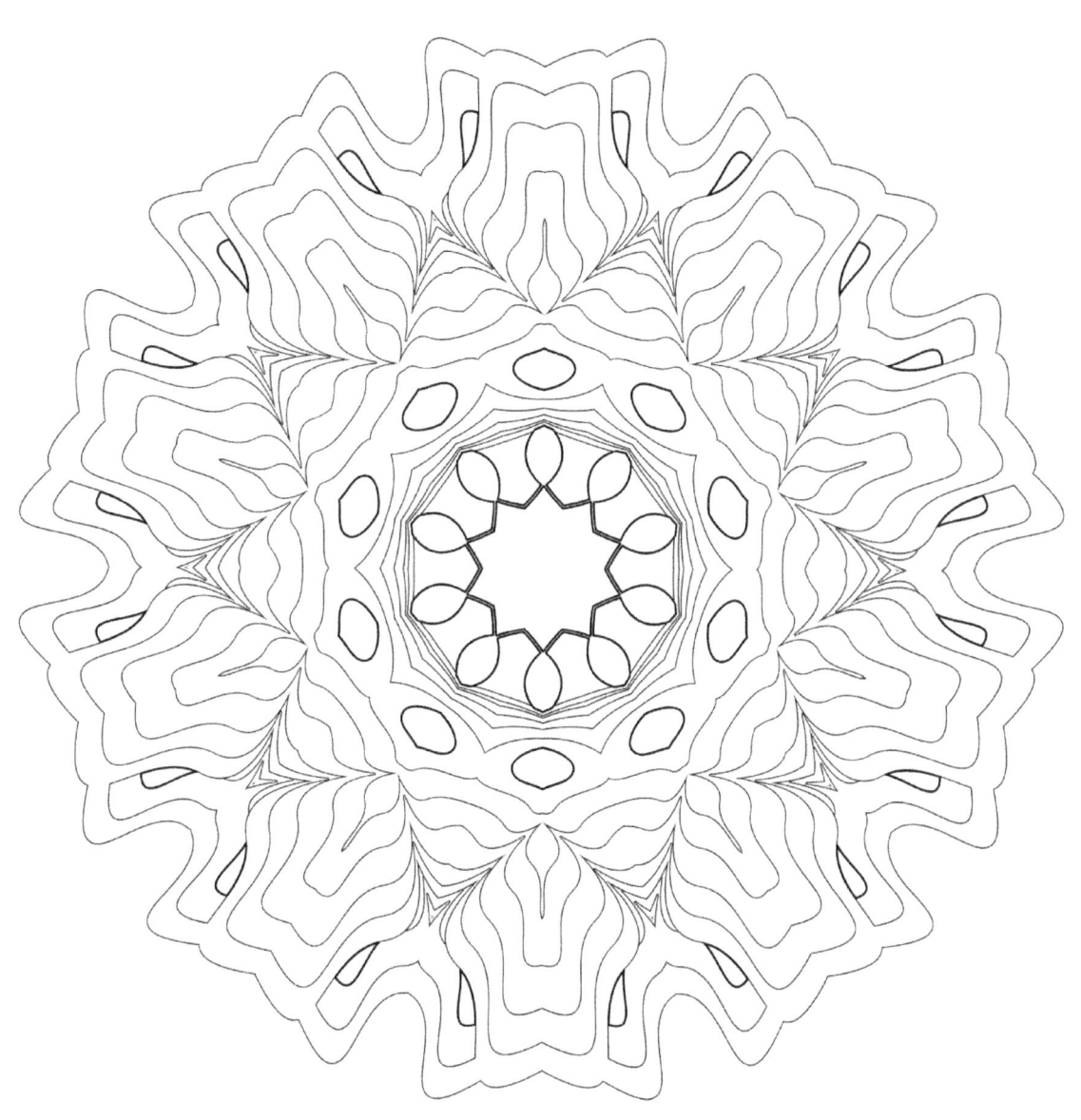

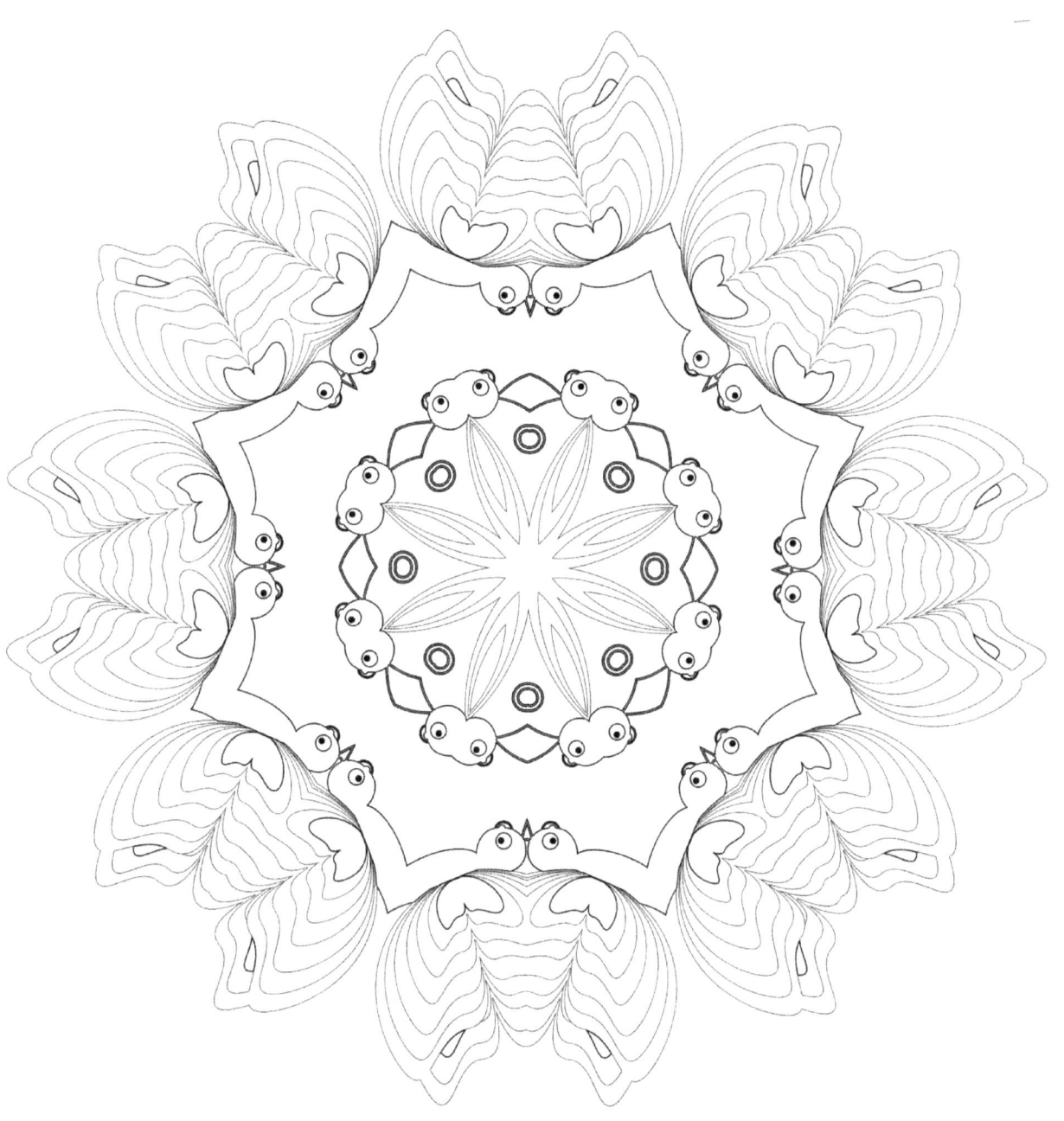

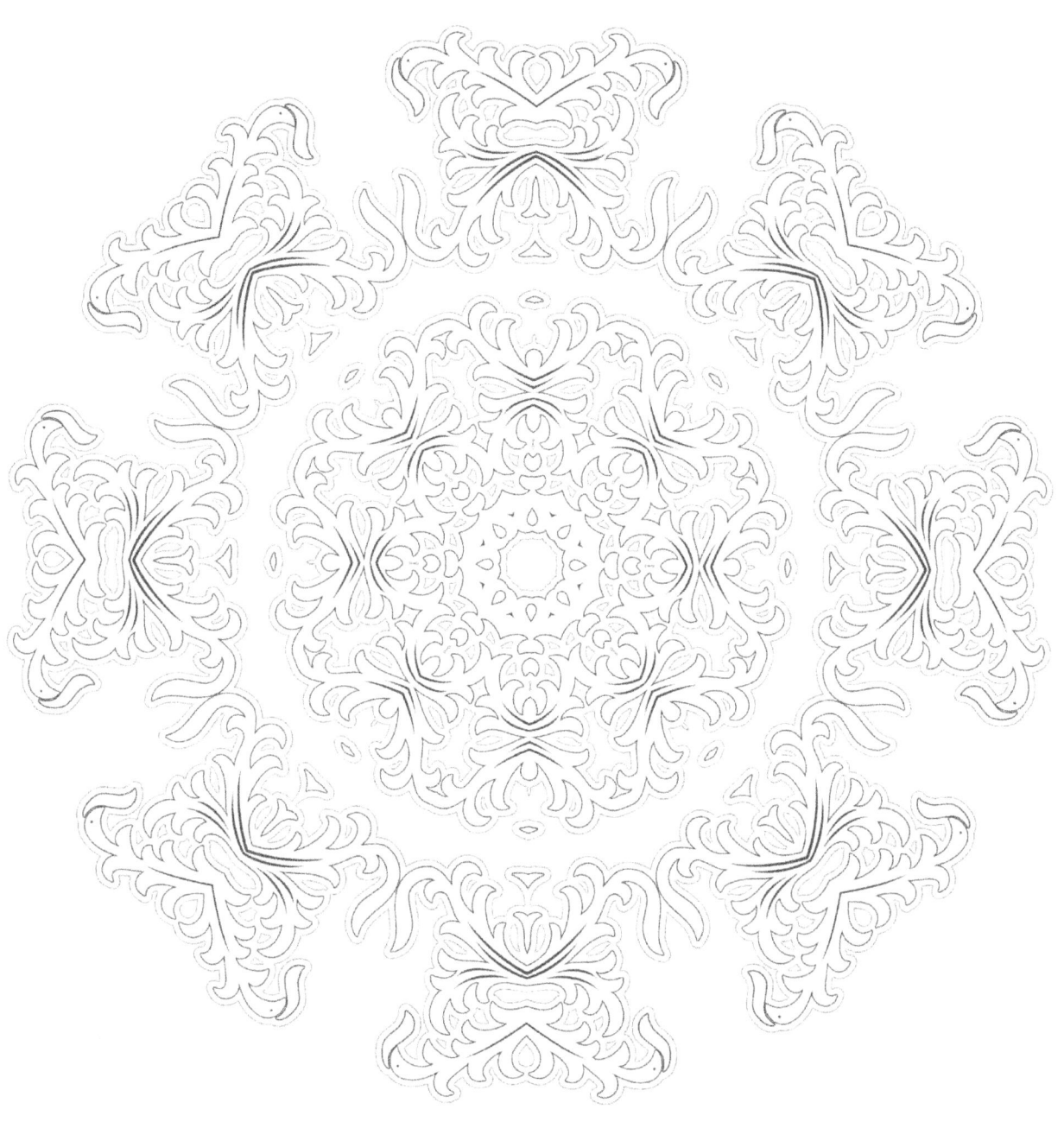

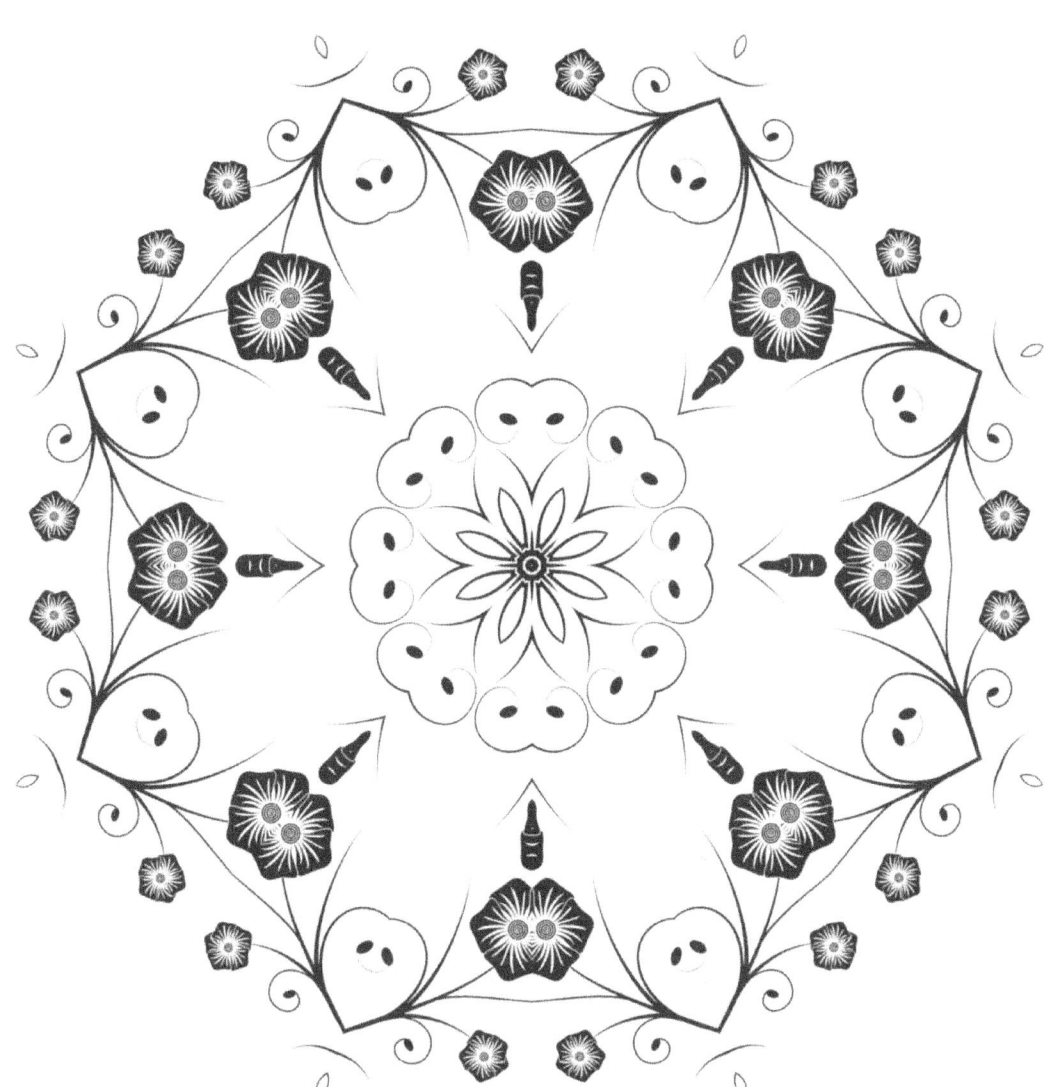

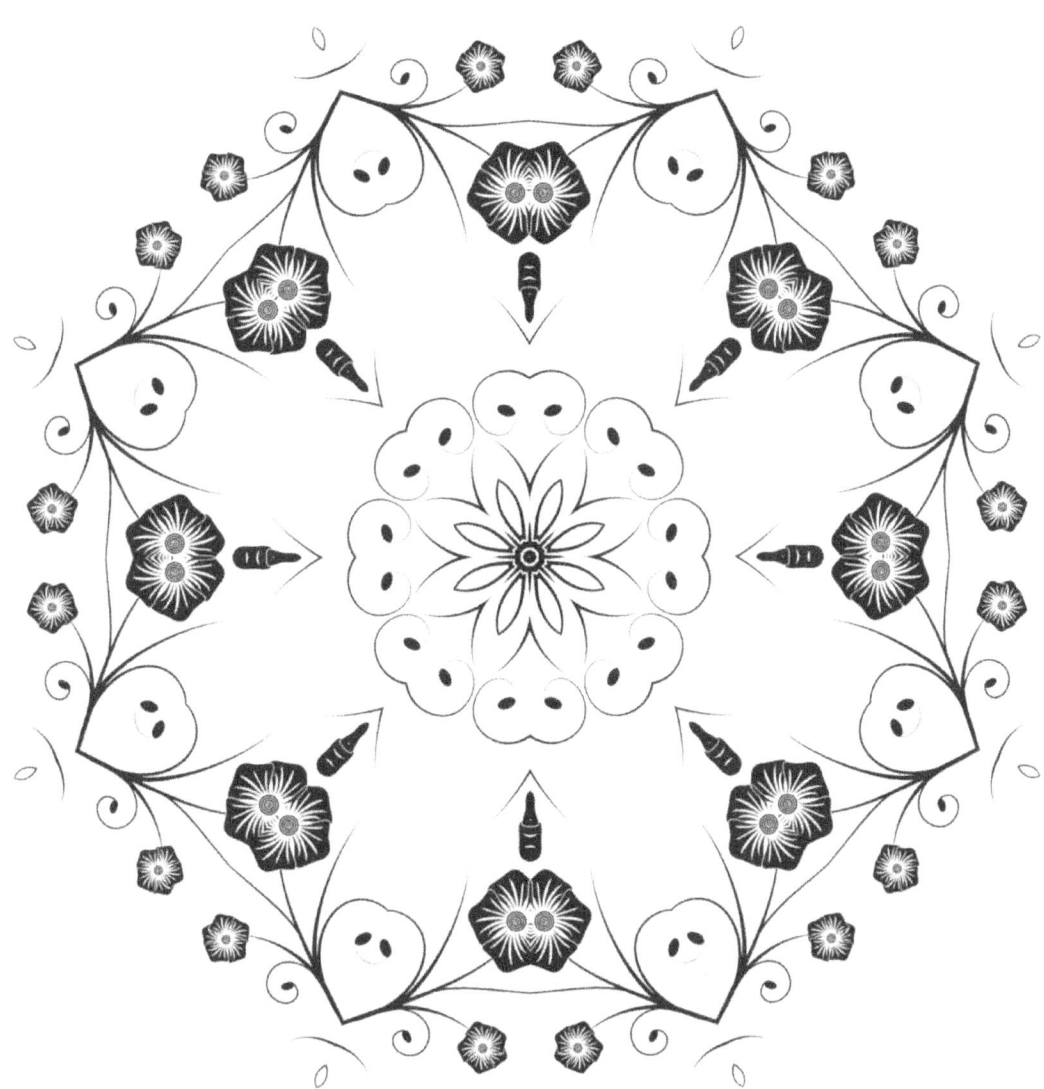

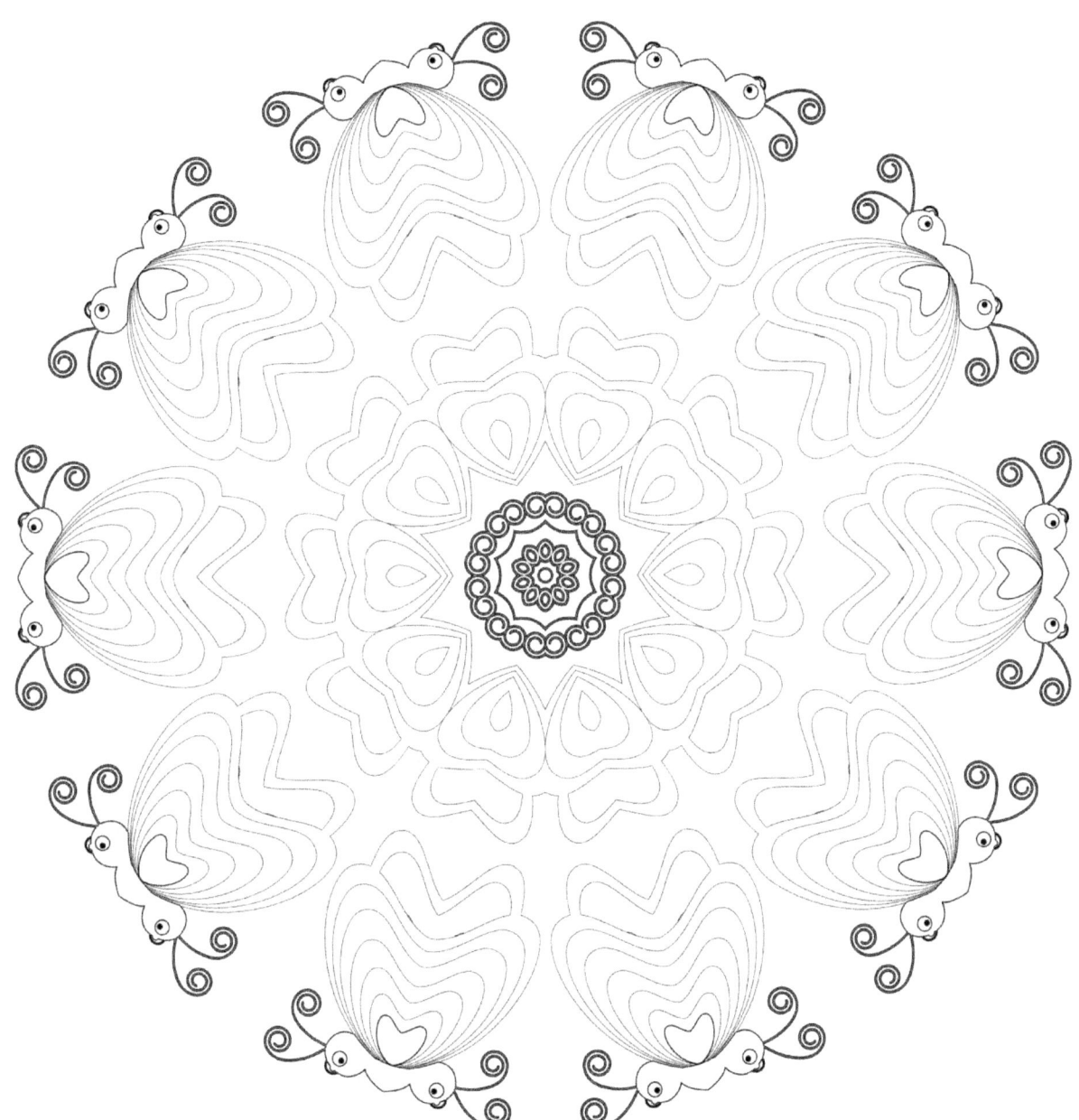

Thank you

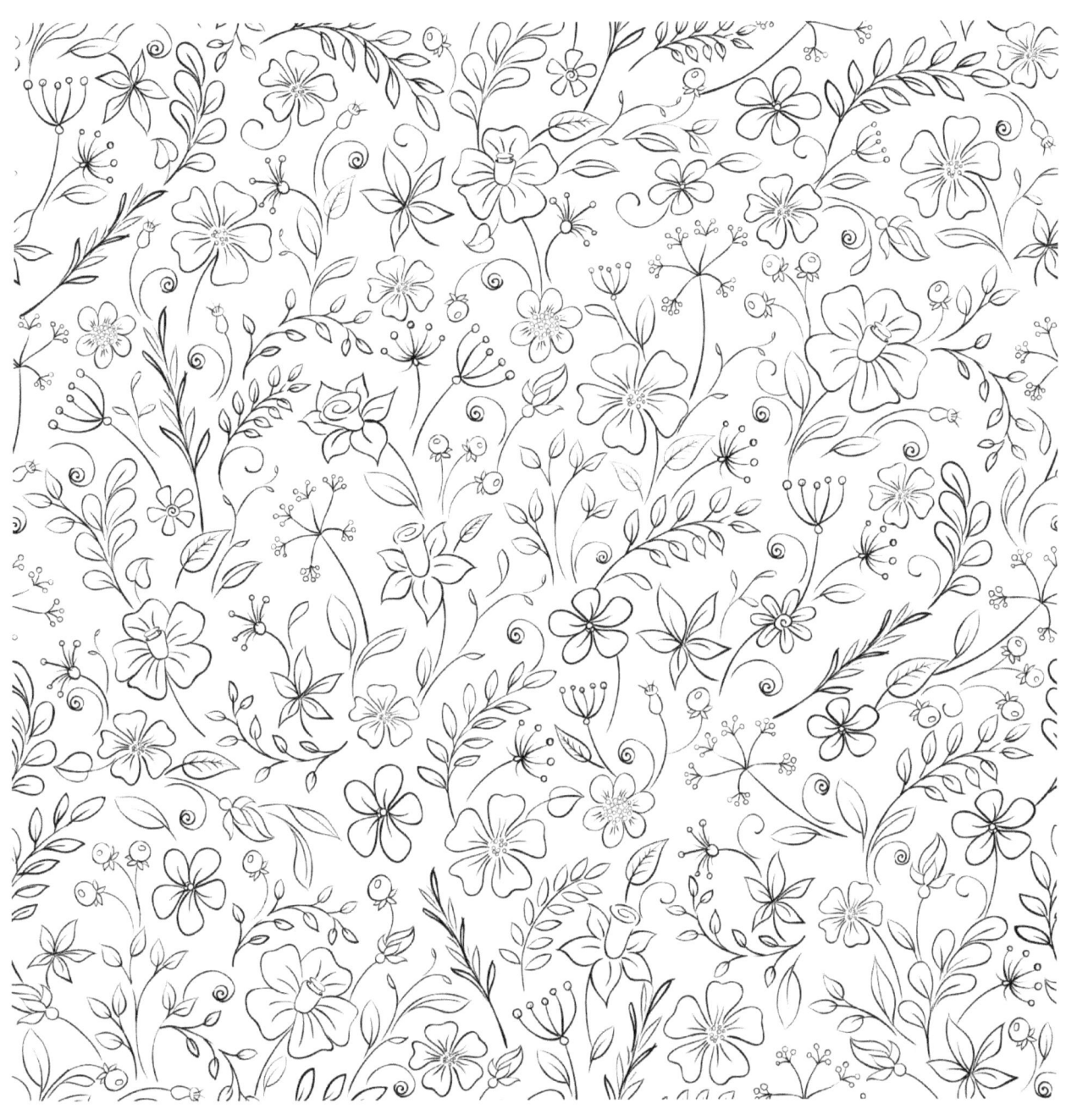